BLOSSOMING BEAUTY

Natural Approaches to Enhance Female Breast Health and Beauty

HAMZA FAGGE AHMAD

Cover design by: Mai Nama Designs
Zoo Road, Kano-Nigeria +2349032351400

CONTENTS

ACKNOWLEDGMENTS

Insert acknowledgments text here. Insert acknowledgments text here.
Insert acknowledgments text here. Insert acknowledgments text here.
Insert acknowledgments text here. Insert acknowledgments text here.
Insert acknowledgments text here. Insert acknowledgments text here.
Insert acknowledgments text here. Insert acknowledgments text here.

CHAPTER 1:
Understanding Breast Health

Breast Anatomy: The Foundation Of Beauty

Understanding the anatomy of the breasts is essential for appreciating the factors influencing their health and appearance. The breast is composed of glandular tissue, fatty tissue, and connective tissue. Glandular tissue includes lobes and ducts responsible for milk production and transportation, while fatty tissue provides shape and support. The intricate network of blood vessels and lymphatic vessels ensures proper circulation and drainage.

Key Concepts:

Lobes and Ducts: Explore the role of lobes and ducts in milk production and the cyclical changes during the menstrual cycle.

Connective Tissue: Understand how connective tissue contributes to breast structure and elasticity.

Hormonal Influences: The Dance Of Estrogen And Progesterone

Hormones, particularly estrogen and progesterone, play a pivotal role in breast development and health. The menstrual cycle orchestrates hormonal fluctuations, influencing breast tenderness, swelling, and overall appearance. Estrogen promotes breast tissue growth, while progesterone contributes to the development of glandular tissue in preparation for potential pregnancy.

Key Concepts:

Menstrual Cycle Phases: Examine the influence of hormonal changes during the menstrual cycle on breast health.

Pregnancy and Lactation: Explore how hormones support breast changes during pregnancy and breastfeeding.

CHAPTER 2:
The Role of Nutrition

Balanced Diet: Nourishing Beauty From Within

A balanced and nutrient-rich diet is fundamental to overall health and well-being, and it plays a crucial role in supporting breast health. A variety of nutrients contribute to the maintenance of healthy breast tissue and hormonal balance. Antioxidants, vitamins, and minerals derived from a colorful array of fruits and vegetables are essential components of a diet that fosters vitality and supports the body's natural processes.

Key Concepts:

Antioxidants: Learn how antioxidants protect cells from damage and may play a role in reducing the risk of breast-related issues.

Omega-3 Fatty Acids: Explore The Benefits Of Omega-3 Fatty Acids Found In Fatty Fish, Flaxseeds, And Walnuts For Hormonal Balance.

Foods For Breast Health: A Culinary Approach

Certain foods offer specific benefits for breast health.

Incorporating these into your diet provides a proactive approach to overall well-being. Broccoli and other cruciferous vegetables contain compounds that may support hormonal balance, while berries contribute antioxidants that protect against oxidative stress.

Key Concepts:

Cruciferous Vegetables: Delve into the potential benefits of broccoli, kale, and Brussels sprouts for breast health.

Berries and Antioxidants: Understand how berries and colorful fruits combat free radicals and promote cellular health.

CHAPTER 3:
Herbal Allies for Breast Health

Traditional Remedies: Wisdom From Nature

Herbs and plants have a long history of traditional use in supporting female reproductive health. From fenugreek seeds to fennel, explore the herbal allies that have been embraced for their potential benefits. Traditional remedies often focus on hormonal balance, lymphatic support, and overall well-being.

Key Concepts:

Fenugreek Seeds: Examine the traditional use of fenugreek seeds for breast health and potential hormonal influence.

Fennel and Anise: Discover how fennel and anise seeds have been historically used to support lactation and hormonal balance.

Herbal Teas And Infusions: Sipping Wellness

Herbal teas and infusions offer a delightful way to incorporate beneficial herbs into your routine. Explore teas such as red clover, which is believed to have phytoestrogenic properties, and dandelion root, known for its potential detoxifying effects.

Key Concepts:

Red Clover Tea: Learn about red clover's reputation as a source of phytoestrogens and its potential impact on hormonal balance.

Dandelion Root Infusion: Discover how dandelion root tea may support liver health and detoxification processes.

CHAPTER 4:
Lifestyle Practices for Breast Care

Exercise For Chest Muscles: Sculpting Strength And Beauty

Incorporating targeted exercises for the chest muscles not only enhances the overall appearance of the breasts but also contributes to strength and posture. Explore exercises like chest presses, push-ups, and pectoral flys that engage the muscles supporting the breasts. Regular exercise promotes blood circulation, ensuring optimal oxygen and nutrient supply to breast tissues.

Key Concepts:

Pectoral Exercises: Dive into effective exercises that specifically target the pectoral muscles for enhanced chest strength.

Posture Awareness: Understand the importance of good posture in maintaining breast support and preventing sagging.

Breast Massage: Nurturing Through Touch

Breast massage is a self-care practice that promotes circulation and lymphatic drainage. Gentle, circular motions may help reduce fluid retention, ease breast tenderness, and enhance overall breast health. This mindful practice encourages women to connect with their bodies, fostering a positive relationship with this intimate aspect of self-care.

Key Concepts:

Lymphatic Drainage: Learn about the role of breast massage in supporting the lymphatic system and reducing congestion.

Self-Examination Techniques: Integrate breast massage with self-examination practices for early detection of changes.

CHAPTER 5:
Mind-Body Connection

Stress And Hormones: Balancing The Internal Symphony

The mind-body connection plays a crucial role in hormonal balance and breast health. Chronic stress can disrupt hormonal harmony, affecting menstrual cycles and overall well-being. Explore stress management techniques such as meditation, yoga, and deep breathing exercises to promote hormonal balance and emotional well-being.

Key Concepts:

Cortisol and Hormones: Understand the impact of stress-induced cortisol on hormonal balance and breast health.

Mindfulness Practices: Embrace mindfulness as a tool for stress reduction and emotional resilience.

Mindful Practices: Radiating Confidence From Within

Mindful practices extend beyond stress reduction, encompassing a holistic approach to self-care. From guided imagery to affirmations, discover techniques that nurture a positive body image and foster self-confidence. Cultivating self-love and acceptance positively influences how one perceives and cares for the body.

Key Concepts:

Body Positivity: Explore mindful practices that encourage a positive body image and appreciation for individual beauty.

Affirmations for Self-Love: Integrate affirmations into daily routines to enhance self-esteem and confidence.

CHAPTER 6: BEAUTY FROM WITHIN

Self-Care Rituals: Nourishing the Soul

Self-care rituals are an integral part of enhancing overall well-being. Explore a range of rituals, from luxurious baths to aromatherapy that promote relaxation and self-nurturing. These rituals contribute to a sense of beauty and vitality that radiates from within.

Key Concepts:

Aromatherapy for Relaxation: Learn about essential oils that promote relaxation and can be incorporated into self-care rituals.

Luxurious Bathing Routines: Explore ways to turn bath time into a rejuvenating and self-nurturing experience.

Wardrobe Choices: Accentuating Natural Beauty

Fashion choices can complement and accentuate the natural beauty of the body. Understand how clothing styles, bra choices, and posture contribute to showcasing the breasts in a way that aligns with personal style and enhances body confidence.

Key Concepts:

Bra Fitting and Support: Discover the importance of proper bra fitting for breast health and appearance.

Fashion Tips: Explore fashion tips that celebrate diverse body shapes and emphasize personal style.

CHAPTER 7: DEBUNKING MYTHS AND REALISTIC EXPECTATIONS

Myths about Breast Growth: Navigating the Truth

Separate fact from fiction by addressing common myths surrounding breast growth. From misconceptions about exercises to beliefs in miracle foods, debunking these myths helps establish realistic expectations. Understanding the natural variability in breast size and shape promotes self-acceptance.

Key Concepts:

Exercise and Breast Size: Clarify the influence of exercise on breast size and shape, dispelling common misconceptions.

Genetic Factors: Explore the role of genetics in determining breast size and why embracing one's natural form is empowering.

Embracing Natural Beauty: A Call To Authenticity

Encourage a shift in perspective toward embracing natural beauty. Celebrate the diversity of body shapes and sizes, recognizing that beauty is not confined to external standards. Empower women to define their standards of beauty and find confidence in their unique attributes.

Key Concepts:

Authenticity and Confidence: Explore stories of women embracing their natural beauty and finding confidence beyond societal expectations.

Self-Love Journey: Encourage a journey of self-love and acceptance that extends beyond physical appearance.

CONCLUSION

It's important to note that breast size is largely determined by genetics and hormones, and there is no guaranteed method for significant and permanent breast enlargement without surgical intervention. However, some people explore natural methods that may help improve the appearance and health of the breasts. It's crucial to approach such methods with realistic expectations, and it's recommended to consult with a healthcare professional before attempting any changes to ensure safety and appropriateness for individual health.

Here are some strategies that some individuals consider for potentially enhancing the appearance of their breasts:

TRY THE FOLLOWING

1. Chest Exercises:

While exercises can't change the size of the actual breast tissue, they can strengthen the muscles underneath, providing some lift and firmness.

Focus on chest exercises like chest presses, push-ups, and pectoral flys to target the muscles supporting the breasts.

2. Nutrient-Rich Diet:

A balanced and nutritious diet supports overall health, including the health of breast tissues.

Include foods rich in antioxidants, vitamins, and minerals. Consider sources of healthy fats like avocados and nuts.

3. Herbal Supplements:

Some herbs are believed to have estrogen-like effects, potentially influencing breast appearance. Examples include fenugreek, fennel, and wild yam.

Consult with a healthcare professional before taking any herbal supplements, as they may interact with medications or have side effects.

4. Massage And Moisturizing:

Regular breast massage may improve blood circulation and lymphatic drainage.

Use moisturizers or oils during massage to maintain skin elasticity.

5. Wearing The Right Bra:

A well-fitted bra can enhance the appearance of the breasts by providing support and lift.

Consult with a professional for a bra fitting to ensure you're wearing the right size.

6. Posture Improvement:

Good posture can contribute to the overall appearance of the chest. Standing tall and having proper alignment can give the illusion of lifted breasts.

7. Weight Management:

Fluctuations in weight can impact breast size. Maintaining a stable, healthy weight may help prevent sagging.

8. Self-Confidence And Acceptance:

Accepting and embracing your body as it is can significantly impact how you perceive your appearance.

Confidence and self-love contribute to an attractive and positive presence.

It's crucial to approach these strategies with caution and be realistic about the potential outcomes. Additionally, individual responses may vary, and what works for one person may not work for another. Surgical options, such as breast augmentation, remain the most effective and permanent method for significant changes in breast size, but they come with associated risks and considerations. Always consult with a healthcare professional before making significant changes to your lifestyle or considering any form of supplementation.

ABOUT THE AUTHOR

Hamza Fagge Ahmad

Is a philanthropist, writer with passion and deep zeal towards human health and development from the beautiful city of Kano in Nigeria.